SECRETS OF THE SUPER FIT

Proven Hacks to Get Ripped Fast Without Steroids or Good Genetics

David de las Morenas
www.HowToBeast.com

Copyright © 2016 Beast Industries LLC
All rights reserved.

ISBN-13: 978-1539899099
ISBN-10: 1539899098

Disclaimer

All attempts have been made to verify the information in this book; however, neither the author nor the publisher assumes any responsibility for errors, omissions, or contrary interpretations of the content within.

This book is for entertainment purposes only, and so the views of the author should not be taken as expert instruction or commands. The reader is responsible for his or her own actions.

This book is not meant to be used, nor should it be used, to diagnose or treat any medical condition. For diagnosis or treatment of any medical problem, consult your own physician. I recommend consulting a doctor to assess and/or identify any health-related issues prior to making any dramatic changes to your diet and/or exercise regime.

Neither the author nor the publisher assumes any responsibility or liability on behalf of the purchaser or reader of this book.

Buyer Bonus

As a way of saying thank you for your purchase, I'm offering a FREE download that's exclusive to my book and blog readers.

It's a proven step-by-step workout routine optimized to quickly pack on mass and get stronger.

Here's what you get inside:

- A complete step-by-step workout routine
- Optimized to build mass in just 3 workouts per week
- All you need is dumbbells and a pull-up bar
- Forced progression means progress is guaranteed
- No guesswork: detailed instructions tell you EXACTLY what to do

...and much, much more.

Download it here now:
http://www.howtobeast.com/get-jacked

Dedication

This book is dedicated to everyone who helped me stay consistent and motivated throughout my entire fitness journey. To my cousin Matt, who introduced me to lifting weights back in college. To the great Alan Aragon, whose kind words encouraged me to keep going after I published my first book. And to all of my personal training clients, who continually challenge me to expand my knowledge and learn new things. Thank you all.

Contents

PROLOGUE: THE "SECRET" TO GETTING RIPPED 1

WHY 99% OF GUYS FAIL TO GET RIPPED 3

HOW I FINALLY TRANSFORMED MY BODY AFTER YEARS OF FRUSTRATION 9

HOW TO USE THIS BOOK FOR MAXIMUM RESULTS 15

PART I: MINDSET HACKS 19

WHAT MOTIVATES YOU? 21

THE HARSH TRUTH 27

LOOK THE PART 35

ACCEPT REALITY 41

SHIFT YOUR PRIORITIES 47

PART II: DIET HACKS 51

YOU'VE BEEN SCAMMED 53

THE TRUTH ABOUT CALORIES 59

COUNTING HACKS 65

SMOKE AND MIRRORS 69

THE SHORTCUT TO GAINS 75

PART III: TRAINING HACKS	81
STOP HOPPING	83
INSTANT GAINS	89
STACK IT UP	93
BREAD AND BUTTER	99
THE TRUTH ABOUT CARDIO	105
RECAP: SECRETS OF THE SUPER FIT	109
YOUR NEXT STEP	113
CAN YOU DO ME A FAVOR?	115
MY OTHER BOOKS	117
ABOUT THE AUTHOR	119
REFERENCES	121

PROLOGUE: The "Secret" to Getting Ripped

Secrets of the Super Fit

Why 99% of Guys Fail to Get Ripped

Let's be honest here: if you're reading this book then you aren't 100% satisfied with your body.

You probably want to build some muscle. And you probably want to cut fat and get leaner, too.

Well, you're not alone. In fact, almost every guy out there is struggling to improve his body. Now, you can take this fact in one of two ways:

- First, you can let yourself off the hook.

Hell, if every other guy is also unhappy with his body, then you might as well just give up, right? Why waste your time?

- Second, you can decide to figure out what the 1% are doing right.

You can realize that every guy who has successfully achieved a ripped body was once in the exact same situation as you. If they figured it out, so can you.

Since you bought this book, I can only assume (and

hope) that you're in the second category. So first off, congrats! Making that simple realization is the first step to transforming your body.

Now, let's get one more thing out of the way. Let's go over what I like to call "the 3 big excuses"…

#1: But aren't they all using steroids?

Yes, okay. Some guys are using steroids. If you do a simple Google image search for "IFBB pro", you will see several hundred images of bodybuilders who are on the juice.

(Side note: the IFBB is a major bodybuilding competition that doesn't test for steroids)

But that's not the look most guys are going for anyway. Most guys want to be lean, muscular, and strong… not look like the freakin' Hulk.

In this book, you'll discover the tools you need to get that lean, muscular look you desire WITHOUT resorting to drug use.

#2: What if I have "bad" genetics?

This is another legitimate concern. Some guys are simply born with an innate advantage.

For example, some guys have naturally broad shoulders that make them look big and strong before they even lift a single weight. And other guys have favorable "muscle insertions". In other words, their muscles are naturally positioned and shaped in a way that looks good (even if they're not very developed).

In this book, you'll learn the tools you need to look great naked regardless of how "bad" your genetics are.

#3: What if I don't have time to work out every day?

This is the last big excuse I hear guys making. But this one is pure BS.

You don't need to work out every day in order to build muscle and burn fat. It's simply a myth.

In fact, your body needs rest days to recover from the stress of lifting weights. So go ahead and scratch this excuse off your list.

(Side note: you can grab my 3-day per week workout routine in the "Buyer Bonus" chapter at the very beginning of this book)

Here's the main point: None of these 3 things are why 99% of guys fail to get ripped.

Nope. It's not that you need steroids. It's not that you have "bad" genetics. And it's not because you don't have time to work out every day...

So what it is then?

It's pretty simple actually: you're focusing on all the wrong things.

Almost every guy is focused on finding the "perfect" diet, the "perfect" workout routine, and the "most effective" supplement regimen. They read fitness article after fitness article, hoping to discover the one "secret" ingredient that will magically transform their body.

Hint: you will never find it.

(Because it doesn't exist)

So what it is? What do the 1% focus on that the other 99% are missing?

Simple. They focus on the basics, every single day, year in and year out. And all of the little, seemingly insignificant progress they make every week – it adds up.

They follow their workout routine consistently. They eat with a purpose. They rinse and repeat.

Just like investing in a retirement account, the results compound over time. And, before you know it, you're jacked!

Now, unfortunately, this is a lot easier said than done.

The real "secret" of the super fit – the one thing

almost all of them have in common – is that they find a way to program themselves to love the process, take action, and follow through on their goals... no matter what life throws at them.

They've all developed a set of special habits that allow them to push forward and stay the course. And they use these things to their advantage, every single day.

The result is consistent, undeniable progress.

In this book, I will reveal the top 15 "secrets" of the super fit – 15 simple hacks, habits, and techniques to program your body for inevitable success. I have discovered these things over years of trial-and-error, research, training, and more.

But wait! Who the hell I am to teach you anything in the first place?

Well, allow me to explain...

How I Finally Transformed My Body after Years of Frustration

If you're skeptical, I totally get it.

There are so many fitness "gurus" these days that you have to be careful.

But before you grab a pitchfork and burn me at the stake, let me introduce myself: my name is David de las Morenas. I'm a personal trainer, certified strength coach, and the founder of **howtobeast.com**...

And while I could brag about how I'm a #1 Men's Health bestselling author, how my blog gets over 100,000 visits per month, or how I've been featured in top fitness publications like *AskMen* and *Bodybuilding.com* – I don't want to waste your time.

I'd rather tell you the story of how I went from a scrawny kid who couldn't get laid to looking like

Captain America (and transforming my entire life in the process)...

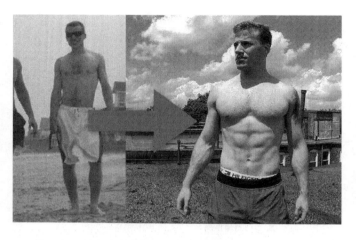

It all started back in college...

After years of playing sports, I got to college and stopped all physical activity. I ate pizza, played video games, and got drunk almost every day.

By the end of my first year, I put on 20 pounds. And all of it was fat. Every time I looked in the mirror, it was painful. I looked like crap. And I lost all confidence in myself.

That summer I was determined to get back in shape. So I followed the typical fitness advice. I started running every day and eating "healthy" foods like salads and smoothies.

My life sucked. I don't even like running. And I was

hungry all the time. But by the end of the summer, I had lost over 40 pounds.

Great, right?

Actually, not so great. I was scrawny as fuck! No joke – I looked like I was starving to death. So I decided to start lifting weights. My cousin recommended P90X: an at-home workout program...

After 1 full year of working out in my basement almost every day, I had nothing to show for it... Okay, maybe my arms grew by like half an inch.

I was so frustrated that I actually stopped working out.

Then, a few months later, I met an amateur bodybuilder and he taught me all about "bulking" and "cutting".

So I started to devour bodybuilding articles online. I decided that I needed to "bulk" up and gain a bunch of weight. I even found a new workout program on bodybuilding.com – I was SO excited to get started!

Fast forward 6 months and I had regained just about all 40 pounds. Sure, I had built some muscle, but I also put on a thick layer of fat. I was literally afraid to take my shirt off around other people.

The frustration was killing me! I dedicated so much time to working out and counting calories – and here

I was, chubby as a donut.

Honestly, I wished I'd just stayed scrawny. It was better than being fat.

So I decided to lose weight again. After 3 months of starvation and cardio, I was skinny as hell… yet again. I truly believed that I was destined to look soft and pudgy forever.

Can you relate to any of this frustration? Have you faced similar obstacles in your fitness journey?

At that point, it felt like I had wasted years of my time trying to make progress, with little-to-no results to show for it. And my self-confidence was at an all-time low because of how I looked.

The good news is that things began to change soon after that. Within the next year, I made more progress than I had made in the prior three years combined. In fact, I was so amped up that I quit my job as a software engineer, got certified, and became a personal trainer.

Not to mention, my self-esteem and motivation skyrocketed in all areas of my life. For the first time ever, I had the courage to approach cute girls and ask them out. I even started dating my first girlfriend!

Over the next few years, I trained hundreds and hundreds of clients. I also continued to build muscle, burn fat, and get stronger myself. And as I went, I discovered more and more "secrets" that allowed me to stay consistent when times got tough, smash through challenging plateaus, and keep making progress year after year...

And these "secrets" had nothing to do with finding the perfect workout routine or eating the latest "superfood"...

No, these "secrets" were simple hacks, habits, and techniques that almost nobody talks about in the world of fitness. They aren't as "sexy" as the hottest muscle-building workout trend, or the latest fat-burning supplement stack.

But they're more important than all of these things combined. They give you the foundation you need to guarantee quick results and steady progress... without steroids, good genetics, or wasting all of your time in the gym.

They are the real reason I was able to make the transformation you saw in the picture at the beginning of this chapter.

...So what are these "secrets"?

Well, keep reading. In this book, I will share my top 15 with you.

Secrets of the Super Fit

How to Use This Book for Maximum Results

Okay, before we get into the "secrets", let me explain the structure of the book. This way, you'll know exactly how to read it and exactly how to apply the techniques inside for maximum impact.

First things first, the book is divided into three main sections:

#1: Mindset Hacks

#2: Diet Hacks

#3: Training Hacks

In the first section, you will learn simple hacks and techniques to change your mindsets regarding fitness. You will learn how to program your mind to take action on autopilot.

This will solve the "motivation problem". In other words, you will no longer need to rely on spurts of motivation or inspiration in order to get your ass to the gym (or eat right). This will allow you to follow through on your goals without even thinking about it.

In the second section, you will learn simple hacks and techniques to optimize your diet for insane muscle growth and fat loss. You will learn the "secrets" to make progress while still enjoying your favorite foods every single day.

Let's get one thing straight: this is not a diet plan. This is simply a set of tools that will allow you to make sure your diet is supporting your fitness goals, without getting lost in some BS fad diet that doesn't do shit for you.

In the final section, you will learn simple hacks and techniques to supercharge your progress in the gym. You will learn key tweaks and tools to make sure you see fast results, regardless of the specific workout routine you're currently using.

Without these things, your progress relies solely upon luck and good fortune.

That being said, it's important to read the book in this order. Your mindsets must be aligned in order for your diet and training to have any lasting effect. And your diet must be optimized if you want your training routine to be as effective as possible.

As you read each chapter, think about how it applies to your life and your gym routine. At the end of each chapter, I have included specific action steps for you to take. Don't ignore these. If you read this book and don't implement the advice, then it will do nothing for you...

But if you *do* take action? This just might be the turning point in your fitness career. It just might be the boost you need to finally take your body to the next level.

Good luck. Let's do this!

PART I: Mindset Hacks

Secrets of the Super Fit

What Motivates You?

"What do you want to accomplish in the gym?"

That is the first question I ask every single one of my personal training clients.

They usually reply: "I want to lose weight." Or maybe: "I want to bulk up and build muscle."

Regardless of their answer, I reply: "Okay cool. WHY do you want to do this?"

I want to know why they're going to the gym in the first place. I want to know what is motivating them to improve their body.

Now, the unfortunate truth is that almost nobody knows the answer to this question – at least not without some additional thought.

In fact, almost every client I've ever trained looks back at me with a blank stare and says: "Uhhh, what do you mean?"

So I try and help them out: "What is your main motivation for reaching this goal?"

At this point, I usually start hearing answers like: "I just want to look better naked" or "I want to be healthier, I guess."

But that's not good enough. That's not the REAL reason that you decided to subject yourself to hours upon hours of working out, sweating, and pushing your body past its limits. No, there's always something deeper.

So I keep pushing. I keep asking "why". Even if it makes them uncomfortable and they start to get defensive. I need to break past the BS and discover their real motivation. And they need to realize it as well.

Eventually, after several minutes of prying, I start to get some answers: "I want to build muscle because I want to be more attractive to girls. I want to get laid. I want a girlfriend."

Or maybe: "I want to get stronger because I'm about to have my first child. I want to be able to play with him and keep up with his energy."

Or maybe: "I want to lose weight because people always crack jokes about how chubby I am. I feel like shit about myself. If I can lose weight, then I'll finally feel worthy of getting respect from my peers."

Damn, shit just got real...

Look, I'm not a therapist. I don't claim to be. But I

know how basic human psychology works. If you're only motivated by vague, external rewards then you won't put in the effort needed to succeed and see results.

If you just want to "get fit" or "burn fat" or "build muscle" then you're doomed to fail. It's simply not enough of a motivator to make you take action and follow through on your goals each and every day of your life.

You need to have some real "skin" in the game. You need to know EXACTLY why improving your body is important to you. Only then will you be able to embrace the daily grind of working out and eating right. Only then will it stop feeling like a chore. Only then will it become something you actually look forward to.

I promise I'm not making this shit up. I can tell you – with complete certainty – that my clients who are able to find a deeper motivation are far more likely to stay consistent, stay committed, and eventually reach their fitness goals.

And the ones who aren't able to think of a deeper motivation? They almost always quit within a few weeks or months. Without knowing your real "why", it's just not worth the effort.

Plus, studies have been done to confirm this psychological fact. For example, one study examined

1,042 students at the University of Quebec in Canada. [1]

All of the students were enrolled in the same class at the beginning of the year. And they all completed an assessment to determine their motivation for taking the course.

At the end of the semester, researchers found that students who were intrinsically motivated to take the course were far more likely stay in the course and earn high marks versus those who took the course simply because they were required to do so or because they needed to earn credits.

In other words, students who took the course because they were actually interested in the material were far less likely to drop out than students who were taking it simply to fulfill a requirement.

While this seems logical, it's still a bit surprising. Even if they were less interested in the course material, you would still expect the second group of students to stay in the course and get the credits they needed. But they didn't. And the ones who did got worse grades.

This proves that your motivations really do matter. If you have a deeper motivation to achieve a goal, you're far more likely to embrace the process, put in the work, and eventually succeed than if you were just doing it to earn some external "reward". You're also more likely to do a better job.

This means that if you can uncover your true motivation for wanting to improve your body, it will be far easier for you to embrace the daily grind of going to the gym, lifting weights, and eating an appropriate diet. It means you will see faster results in the short term, and better results in the long term.

Now it's your turn...

Right now, take a few minutes to determine your "deeper" motivation for improving your body.

- Start by getting clear on your main goal: exactly what do you want to accomplish in the gym?
- Then, ask yourself: why do you want to accomplish this?
- Repeat that step, ask yourself "why" five times in total.

Let's run through a hypothetical example, so you can see what I mean:

What do I want to accomplish in the gym? I want to see my six pack and build more muscle.

Why do I want to accomplish this? Because I want to look better naked.

Why do I want to look better naked? Because I want girls to think I'm better looking.

Why do I want girls to think I'm better looking? Because I want to date more women.

Why do I want to date more women? Because I want to find a cool girlfriend.

Why do I want to find a girlfriend? Because I want someone to create and share awesome experiences with.

...And now you know your deeper motivation. Now you're not working out just to "see your six pack". Instead, you're working out to find a loving girlfriend to share experiences with.

Just making this realization will increase your drive to stay consistent with your workouts and your diet. It will make you far more likely to succeed in achieving your goals.

Now, that's just an example. There are no right or wrong answers here.

One last note: don't expect this process to be easy. It may take some digging and internal reflection before you get to the fourth or fifth "why".

Just be patient with yourself. It's worth the effort.

The Harsh Truth

What is your goal body?

Think about that for a second. If I asked you to find a picture of someone's body you'd like to have, who would you select?

For most guys, they would say one of three things:

"I want to look like that actor in the latest superhero movie. The wolverine is freaking ripped!"

"That running back on the Dallas Cowboys is jacked as hell! That's what I want to look like."

"Dude, this one guy on Instagram is shredded to pieces! I wonder what his secret is…"

It's easy to look at movie stars, professional athletes, and fitness models for inspiration. You know, guys who have the type of body you see on a magazine cover. They give you something to aim for.

Now, I hate to be the bearer of bad news, but the harsh truth is that A LOT of these guys are using steroids. Before you write me off as a hater, take a minute to hear me out…

I'll start by providing some proof that steroid use is

very prevalent these days. And then I'll explain how you can use this knowledge to your advantage (and avoid a common trap that can destroy your progress in the gym).

Let's start with professional athletes. Most people assume that because they are tested for steroids, they don't use them. This is a very naïve belief. The fact is that steroid development is far ahead of drug testing procedures. In other words, it's very easy for athletes to "cheat" the tests.

For proof of this, look no further than the infamous Lance Armstrong case. He literally passed HUNDREDS of drug tests over his 15+ year career as the world's best cyclist, only to later admit to using steroids and other PEDs (performance enhancing drugs) almost the entire time.

There was even one testimony in his case that described when he passed a drug test, all because he was given a mere 5 MINUTES notice. That's all the time he needed to inject saline into his blood stream, effectively diluting his urine and allowing him to pass the test. [2]

If that's not enough proof, consider the fact that professional athletes have come forward in nearly every major sport confirming the use of steroids. Here are a few examples:

- Jose Canseco, former pro baseball player, stated

that "over 80%" of the MLB uses steroids [3]
- Derek Rose of the Chicago Bulls said that steroid use is a "huge" problem in the NBA [4]
- Eddie George, former NFL running back, said that PED use is "very prevalent" in football [5]

The burning question, of course, is: how can all this be true? Why do so many guys put their health in jeopardy and use steroids?

The answer is quite obvious. As soon as one guy starts taking steroids, he gains an advantage. Other players realize this, and they're "forced" to do the same. They have to... at least if they want to remain competitive.

And let's be honest: professional athletes are the most competitive people in the world. Plus, their paycheck depends on them being the best at what they do. They have an intense motivation to succeed, and this makes them liable to bend the rules, if necessary.

The same is true for movie stars who are competing to secure the lead role in the latest superhero movie. The same is true for the hordes of fitness models who are trying to get noticed by top photographers and supplement companies.

Hell, I've been offered steroids multiple times in my life, without ever going out of my way to express any interest in them. I even know former college athletes that were regularly injected by their trainers.

For the better or worse, steroid use has become extremely common in our society today.

So why is this so important? And how can it actually help you achieve your fitness goals?

I'm glad you asked. I was starting to rant there.

It's pretty simple actually. By realizing that the top tier of bodies you see on a daily basis are a result of probable drug use, you can adjust your expectations.

No, I'm not telling you to give up your fitness goals, lie down on the couch, and start stuffing your face in misery. You can still naturally achieve an awesome body that turns heads and drops panties...

But you're never going to look like your favorite Instagram model or pro football player – not without using steroids at least.

This is such an important realization to make because a lot of guys give up and quit when they fail to see the immediate results they've been led to believe are possible. Rather than staying consistent, putting in the hard work, and seeing some great results over time, they get demoralized and give up after only a few months of working out.

By adjusting your aim, and setting realistic expectations, you can greatly increase the likelihood of following through on your goals and achieving a great body.

It's not going to happen overnight. It might not even happen in the next couple months. But if you stay consistent in the long run, then you WILL build a ripped body you can be proud of.

So... exactly what are REALISTIC expectations?

Let's dive in.

Lyle McDonald, one of the top bodybuilding researchers, constructed a simple model for what we can expect in terms of natural muscle growth, based on how long we've been training. [6]

It looks like this:

Year of Proper Training	Potential Rate of Muscle Gain per Year
1	20-25 pounds (2 pounds per month)
2	10-12 pounds (1 pound per month)
3	5-6 pounds (0.5 pound per month)
4+	2-3 pounds (not worth calculating)

In other words, the amount of muscle you can build decreases as you build more and more muscle. At first, you can build as much as 2 pounds per month. But several years down the line, it's a lot less than that.

Now, these numbers aren't set in stone. But they are

an accurate representation of what most guys should expect.

This means you should stop expecting to make a transformation like this one:

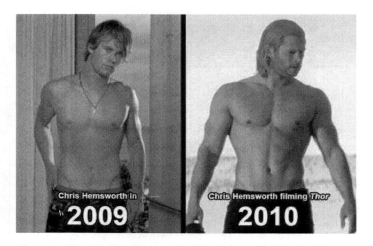

And instead expect something more like this:

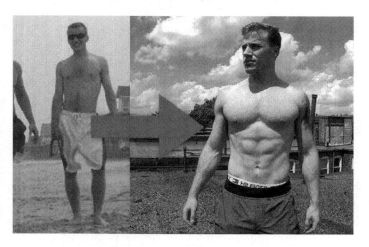

That first shot is a 1-year progress photo of actor Chris Hemsworth. The end result is not completely unattainable, just not attainable in a single year (without the help of drugs).

The second shot is a 4-year transformation photo of myself. This is by no means the ceiling of what you can expect, but it's an example of what four years of consistency can bring you (as well as a big tattoo on your arm).

Again, you can 100% achieve a lean, muscular body that's better than 99% of guys out there. But, unless you take steroids, you shouldn't expect to transform your body overnight.

Keep this in mind as you go forward. It will save you useless frustration and self-doubt that might otherwise convince you to quit working out and give up on achieving an awesome body.

Secrets of the Super Fit

Look the Part

What gym do you go to? And what do you usually wear to the gym?

These two questions might seem trivial – and a bit random – but they actually play a large role in your fitness results.

You see, most of us are cheap people. Sure, you may have a few vices where you like to splurge, but on average you probably do your best to constrain your spending.

Maybe you're like me and you have a soft spot for eating out. Boy, how those dinner bills can quickly add up. Or maybe you have an expensive hobby like cycling, golfing, or fishing.

Either way, you probably feel comfortable spending money on certain areas of your life, but not others. This is only natural.

In fact, studies show that we are much more risk averse to spending money than spending time. We would rather waste several hours of time trying to figure something out than spending a few hundred dollars to get help. [7]

So, why is this important when it comes to working

out and seeing results?

Well, it's pretty straightforward: if you invest money into your fitness habit, you're more likely to stay consistent and follow through on your goals. Let's dive in a bit deeper, because I know you may be skeptical here.

In general, there are two areas where I would advise making calculated investments in your body: the clothes you work out in and the gym you go to.

First, let's talk gym clothes.

Do you think it's a coincidence that nearly every girl you see wearing Lululemon yoga pants is in great shape?

(Side note: Lululemon is an expensive fitness brand, known for women's yoga clothing. Their yoga pants cost more than $100 per pair.)

Studies show that the way we dress actually impacts how we feel and how we perform. For example, one study examined the effects of wearing a superhero t-shirt. And its findings were pretty shocking.

"When wearing a Superman t-shirt the students rated themselves as more likable and superior to other students. When asked to estimate how much they could physically lift, those in a Superman t-shirt thought they were stronger than students in a plain t-shirt, or in their own clothing."

The shocking part is that they also experienced a boost in performance. On mental ability tests, participants wearing the superhero shirts scored an average of 72%, whereas those wearing plain t-shirts scored an average of 64%. [8]

In other words, wearing certain clothes can change how you see yourself. And these changes can actually improve your performance.

So how do you use this to increase your results in the gym?

Basically, just buy fresh clothes that get you excited to hit the gym. Think about it this way: would you rather step into the gym in some sweatpants from the 90s and an old high school t-shirt, or a fresh new outfit that enhances your physique and keeps you cool and dry?

Unless you're an old school bodybuilder, who's addicted to working out in hilariously ancient clothing, I'm guessing you picked the second option.

Not only will you physically feel more comfortable while you're at the gym, you'll also look like you're in better shape. Plus, the act of spending money on gym clothes will increase your investment in working out. And all of this will combine to get you more excited to hit the gym, and maybe even perform better while you're there.

I'm not going to sell you hard on any one brand here,

but workout clothes have come a long way in the past 10 years. They fit better, making your body appear more jacked. And they work better, too, in terms of wicking away sweat and having a bit of stretch to avoid constraining your movement when you're trying to hit that deep squat. Anything new from Nike or Lululemon (yes, they also make men's clothes) is a good place to start.

Now, I also believe you should consider investing in a membership at a high-quality gym.

Again, the mere act of spending money on fitness will increase your likelihood of staying consistent and following through, because we all inherently hate wasting money. If you spend $100 per month on a membership at a luxury gym like Equinox or Life Time Fitness, you're more likely to show up than if you were only spending $20 per month at a run-down facility. You simply don't have much to lose if you decide not to go.

Trust me, I worked as a trainer for years at Equinox. Just about every one of their members is a "regular". They all show up, day after day, and keep putting it work. Now, I've also been a member at low-end gyms like the YMCA and other local chains. And, when you go to these places, it seems like there are new faces there every day. The reality is that most of these "new faces" are actually long-time members, they just only show up once every few weeks.

And, as a result, the members at higher-level gyms tend to be in way better shape. Unfortunately, I don't have a study to quantify this for you, but just take a tour of your local luxury gym and you'll see what I'm talking about.

(Side note: they also have way nicer equipment. Even if you're just doing the basics, deadlifting on a nice platform with real Olympic bars is something you just don't get at low-end gyms.)

Anyway, let's wrap up this chapter.

Spending money on your fitness habit is an investment in your body. It's like making a commitment to yourself. It's like saying, "I'm serious about this shit, so I'm going to put my money where my mouth is."

It will make you more consistent. And this will have a HUGE impact on your results over time. Plus, you'll get to enjoy some awesome perks like super-comfortable clothing, top-of-the-line equipment, and showers that don't look like you're going to catch an STD on the way out.

Obviously, be smart here. If dropping a few hundred dollars on gym clothes means you can't eat for the month, then don't do it. But *do* analyze your expenses and see if you can re-allocate money you're spending on something else (like booze or video games) towards your fitness habits.

Accept Reality

What part of your body are you most embarrassed about?

All of us have insecurities. Sure, women get a bad rap here. We all know horror stories of girls with anorexia or bulimia. But guys aren't immune to these issues either.

In fact, there are a few things that men tend to be SUPER insecure about: being short, having a small penis, looking chubby with your shirt off, looking "small" at the gym, and balding, just to name a few.

Do any of these apply to you?

Don't be ashamed, man. We all have things that we're embarrassed about.

And here's the kicker: the more you focus on your insecurities, and the more you try to "hide" them from other people, the more and more power they gain over you.

I'm going to get real with you here and share a short story from my life.

When I first got into fitness, all I wanted was to build muscle and "get big". I had been relatively scrawny all my life and it made me feel inferior to jacked guys at the gym (and my college buddies who were bigger than me).

On one hand, this gave me an intense motivation to succeed. I was obsessed with working out, counting calories, and looking at myself in the mirror. All I wanted to do was lift weights, eat, and gain weight...

But regardless of how much weight I gained, I was never satisfied. I still felt small. I still felt weak. I still felt like I needed to get bigger in order to be "worthy" of getting respect from other guys (and attracting girls into my life).

And while this did lead me to make a lot of progress in the gym — bulking up from 145 pounds all the way up to about 185 pounds — it crippled my self-esteem in the process. I was always looking around and comparing myself to other guys...

"I wonder how much he can bench press?"

"I bet I look better than him with my shirt off..."

"Is that girl his girlfriend? I could never get a girl like that."

Despite the fact I was improving my body, I was destroying just about every other part of my life. In fact, I stuffed my face with so much Ben & Jerry's ice cream (and numerous other high calories foods, dairy foods — despite the fact I'm lactose intolerant), that I began to experience terrible digestion problems.

I was in the bathroom for ridiculous amounts of time every single day, and I usually felt bloated or sick when I was not. And all of this led me to develop some chronic gastrointestinal health problems (which I just so happened to finally get surgery for earlier this year).

...All in the quest to "get big" and prove my self-worth as a man.

It turns out that this compulsion to build muscle – and the accompanying belief that you're never big enough – is a clinically diagnosable body image issue. It's known as muscle dysmorphia, or bigorexia, and it affects a lot of guys out there. And while it led to some short-term results in the gym, it ultimately caused my body – and my self-confidence – a lot more harm than it was worth.

And the sad thing is that these issues NEVER get discussed in the world of men's health.

The bright side of this story is that I learned a powerful lesson: accepting reality. When I was forced to stop gaining weight, because of the intense digestive pains I was experiencing, I finally realized just how obsessed I had become.

After realizing this, and sharing it with some close friends, everything changed.

"I'm not as big as I want to be. But that's okay. I'll work to get there still, but I won't put my health and well-being on the line in the process," I told myself.

Sure, I lost some weight and lost some of my "gains" at first, but my self-confidence shot through the roof. I had finally accepted reality. I had finally accepted one of my biggest insecurities. And the stranglehold it had taken on my self-esteem quickly faded.

I immediately felt happier and more confident in myself. I immediately began getting out of my comfort zone and doing more than just lifting weights and watching fitness videos on YouTube. And it's no coincidence I also started meeting (and dating) more women than ever before.

Plus, it's been a lot easier to stay consistent in the gym now that I don't feel like I'm "fixing" myself when I'm there. And I enjoy my workouts a whole lot more. It's been about 2 years since I made this mindset shift, and now I'm bigger, leaner, and stronger than ever before.

Sure, that's a nice story. But how can you use this information to your advantage?

Simple. You need to identify and accept your insecurities. Otherwise, they will undermine all of your efforts to improve yourself.

You will be acting from a place of weakness and feeling "unworthy" rather than a place of strength and self-love. And this will cripple your ability to stay consistent in the long-term and see sustainable results.

Start by thinking of everything that you're embarrassed about. What do you hide from other people? What are you secretly ashamed of?

Remember the list from above: height, weight, hairline, penis size, muscle mass, body fat, etc.

Write down anything that comes to mind. The simple process of identifying these things will immediately help remove the power they have over you.

Beyond that, I recommend picking one of your insecurities and sharing it with a close friend. This will be intimidating, but it will be extremely effective in terms of overcoming the damage this thing has done to your self-confidence over the years.

The gym should be a place you go to experience self-growth and a physical "high", not somewhere you go to "fix" yourself.

Shift Your Priorities

How many hours do you sleep on an average night?

If you're like most guys, then your answer is probably 5 or 6 hours.

It can be challenging to get to bed with enough time to get a full 7 or 8 hours of sleep. Maybe you really want to watch the next episode of *Game of Thrones*. Maybe you really need to answer a few more emails. Maybe you're out at the bar with your buddies and you don't want to go home yet.

So you stay up an extra hour or 2... even if it means only sleeping 4 or 5 hours that night.

How does this affect your body – and your ability to build muscle and burn fat?

Well, first of all, is that fact that you'll be tired tomorrow. You will have lower levels of energy and focus all day long, even if you load up on coffee every few hours.

Not that you need anything more than your experience to confirm this fact, but countless studies have been done that show sleep deprivation causes significant decreases in mental abilities and reaction times. [9]

This means you'll be more likely to skip the gym altogether, and even if you do work up the energy to show up, your performance will be comprised. You won't be at your peak strength levels. And this will directly impact your ability to build new muscle and improve your body.

And if this wasn't enough to convince you about the importance of sleep, consider this: many studies have shown that sleep restriction has a HUGE impact on testosterone levels. A recent study measured a 10-15% drop in daytime testosterone levels in healthy young men who underwent one week of sleeping only 5 hours per night. [10]

That's a significant drop!

And many other studies have confirmed the same thing: your total sleep time is a strong predictor of your testosterone levels.

This can severely limit your ability to pack on muscle and burn fat. You see, testosterone plays a key role in muscle protein synthesis: the process by which your body builds new muscle mass. If your testosterone levels are compromised, then so is your ability to build muscle.

And, if you're focused on losing weight, it means your body is far more likely to shed muscle along with fat as you drop the pounds. In other words, you're more likely to end up skinny fat.

And that's not even the worse part. Low testosterone can also lead to a compromised sex drive, decreased sperm production, and lower bone density, just to name a few things.

So, now I hope you can clearly see how important getting sufficient sleep is. If you want to achieve a ripped body that turns heads, you NEED to make it a priority.

Everybody knows how important diet and training is, but sleep is something that all-too-often gets completely overlooked. This makes it one of the biggest predictors of success. It sets apart the 1% of guys who are able to make amazing transformations from the hordes of wannabe's who can never seem to see any results in the mirror.

Look, there will always be something else you can spend your time doing at night. There will always be one more reason to delay your bedtime by another 30 minutes. However, you must put sleep first.

Get your work done earlier in the day. If you can't sleep in, then don't go out late. And, no matter how big of a cliffhanger that Netflix episode ended on, you're going to have to wait until tomorrow to see what happens next.

So exactly how much sleep do I need to get?

Well, there's no magic number here, but I recommend getting 8 hours of uninterrupted sleep per night if you want to ensure that you feel great and that your testosterone levels don't take a hit.

If you struggle to sleep well, here are a few things that have helped me:

- Make sure your room is cool (use AC or leave a window cracked)
- Use a fan to drown out any noise that might wake you up
- Darken your room as much as possible (blackout blinds can help)
- Don't have caffeine at least 6 hours before bedtime
- Avoid stressful or exciting activities for 2 hours before bedtime

It's not the end of the world if you only get 6 hours of sleep every once in a while, just don't make a habit of it.

PART II: Diet Hacks

Secrets of the Super Fit

You've Been Scammed

What diets have you tried in the past?

Chances are, if you're like most guys, you've experimented with one or two diets at some point in your life.

If not, then I'm sure you've at least heard of popular diets like Paleo, Atkins, Slow Carb, or Keto. For all of these diets – and every other diet out there – you can find people who absolutely love them, and people who failed to see any results while using them.

Here's the thing: all diets are "products" by nature. All of them are used to sell you books, programs, and foods. Not only that, but every diet has "experts" who are trying to sell you on the diet itself. They want you to "buy in" to their way of doing things and become one of their fans.

Now, this is not bad or evil per se. Some products out there are useful. Some products add legitimate value to your life. Hell, I have an amazing bed that improves my quality of sleep. I have some amazing workout clothes that improve my experience at the gym. I also have this amazing protein powder that tastes like cinnamon rolls...

But I digress.

The issue here is that diets are not something that should be "sold" to other people. We are all different. We all have different health goals. We all have different food preferences. Our stomachs and digestive systems react differently to different types of foods.

There is no such thing as a one-size-fits-all diet.

To prove this to you, let's take a look at something that's shared by many popular diets: the restriction of carbohydrates. Everything from Paleo and Slow Carb to Atkins and Keto requires you to avoid large groups of carbohydrates.

Why has the idea of restricting carbs gained so much popularity?

Because people often lose 5-10 pounds within a week or 2 of getting started!

But hold up...

The reason for this initial drop in weight is because after your body digests carbs, it stores them in your body as something called glycogen. Now, glycogen is not bad. It's not body fat. In fact, it's actually a primary source of energy for your body during intense bouts of exercise.

Now here's the key fact: glycogen is 3-4 parts water. This means that when you restrict your carb intake, your glycogen stores get emptied, and you lose a bunch of water weight as a result.

In other words, you didn't lose any "real" weight (aka fat), just a bunch of water weight.

Plus, you lose all of your glycogen stores in the process. This will deplete your energy, make you weaker in the gym, and cripple your ability to get stronger and build muscle.

Not to mention, restricting carbs also decreases your testosterone levels.

A recent study performed on two groups of athletes confirms this fact. One group ate a high carb diet (60% of total calories) and the other ate a low carb diet (30% of total carbs). After three days of intense training, the high-carb group had a significantly higher (+43%) ratio of testosterone to cortisol. [11]

Why do I tell you all of this?

Because if you're a guy who wants to get jacked and pack on mass in the gym, then following any of these popular low carb diets will act directly against your goals.

Okay, I get it, it doesn't make sense to follow a low

carb diet. What should I do instead?

Good question.

By now, I hope you can see why every diet out there is essentially a "scam". Not a scam in the sense that people are intentionally trying to trick you and deceive you. But a scam in the sense that they are being advertised as the "best way to eat" when, in reality, they are not.

Instead, you should follow your own diet. Personally, I follow the "David de las Morenas Diet".

I eat 3 big meals per day because it allows me to control my hunger. I don't eat late at night because it makes my stomach feel bloated in the morning. I avoid sugary foods and fried foods during the day because they kill my energy levels (but I still enjoy them at night when I don't have any work left to do). I don't eat dairy foods because I'm lactose intolerant and they make me feel like crap. Other than that, I just make sure to eat enough calories to gain a little bit of weight, because I'm currently focused on gaining mass.

Sure, that's a bit simplified. But the point is that you need to adjust your diet based on YOUR goals, YOUR preferences, and how YOUR body reacts to different foods. Nobody can tell you what's best for you. Because nobody but you can actually feel the effects of what you eat.

Okay, that all sounds good, but what the hell am I actually supposed to do?

Just follow these simple steps to get started with your own diet:

- Eat the right amount of overall calories (we'll go over this in the next chapter)
- Eat a balance of fats, carbs, and protein
- Avoid eating foods that make you feel bad (bloated, tired, etc)
- Make sure the majority of your diet is whole foods (a small amount of "junk" foods is fine)
- Eat whenever you prefer (some people feel better on 3 meals per day, some people prefer 5-6 smaller meals, and some people like to intermittent fast and have only 2 meals)

These guidelines are intentionally vague! Only you can figure out what diet is best for you. The point of this chapter is to get you to WAKE THE FUCK UP and realize that only you can figure out what foods are best for you...

At least if you want to feel good and see fast results in the gym.

The key is to be mindful and notice how your body reacts to different food types, meal sizes, and meal times.

For example, if you feel tired and lazy every time you eat a big lunch, then you shouldn't do that. Or if you feel bloated every time you eat pizza or ice cream, then you should probably stop eating dairy foods.

The Truth about Calories

How much do calories really matter?

This is a topic that gets discussed a lot. It's quite controversial actually. Although I'm still not sure exactly why.

Your caloric balance determines whether you lose, gain, or maintain your weight.

If you eat more calories than you burn, you gain weight. If you eat fewer calories than you burn, you lose weight. It really is that simple.

It's the first law of thermodynamics: energy cannot be created or destroyed. And a calorie is simply a measure of energy. It measures the energy content of food and the amount of energy expended by human beings. [12]

In other words, any extra energy you consume, beyond what your body needs to function, must get stored somewhere. And it either gets stored as glycogen (as discussed in the previous chapter) or as body fat.

And vice versa, all energy your body uses has to come from somewhere. If you don't eat enough food to supply this energy, then you will empty your glycogen stores or burn body fat to make up for the difference.

Anyway, enough of all the scientific BS...

Let's make one thing clear though, the statement that "a calorie is a calorie" is simply not true. Sure, all calories are equal if we're only looking at weight loss or weight gain, but as we explored in the previous chapter, different foods affect your body in different ways.

Some foods are going to affect your energy levels and hunger levels in different ways than others. Some foods are going to give you an upset stomach. 500 calories of French fries is going to make you feel a lot different than 500 calories of chicken.

You can't just eat all of your calories in donuts and candy bars and expect to feel good and see good results in the gym.

That being said, you ABSOLUTELY MUST eat the correct amount of overall calories if you want to efficiently build muscle and burn fat. If you don't, your progress in the gym is going to be severely limited.

There's simply no point in worrying about anything else until your calories are on point. The amount of protein you eat is secondary to eating the right amount of calories. The supplements you take are also secondary.

Hell, even your gym routine is secondary to eating the right amount of calories. You can work your ass off in the gym and still fail to build muscle if you're not eating enough calories. Likewise, you can work your ass off in the gym and still fail to burn fat if you're eating too many calories.

Let's examine that last paragraph a little deeper...

If your goal is building muscle, you need to eat enough calories to gain weight. Why? Because your body needs extra energy in order to synthesize new muscle tissue. It's like having a builder make you a new house. He needs materials like wood, nails, and paint to build it. He can't fabricate it out of thin air. And neither can your body.

Sure, your workouts also need to be on point. But we'll get into that in Part III.

Likewise, if your goal is getting lean, you need to restrict how many calories you eat every day. You need to eat fewer calories than you burn. If you don't, it doesn't matter how hard you train in the gym, your body will have no reason to burn fat.

Okay, so EXACTLY how many calories should I be

eating?

Well, before I answer that question we need to go over how fast you should be aiming to lose or gain weight, because this dictates how many calories your body needs.

When it comes to gaining weight and building muscle, you have to remember that your body has natural limits. As we explored in Part I, your body can only add so much muscle per month:

Year of Proper Training	Potential Rate of Muscle Gain per Year
1	20-25 pounds (2 pounds per month)
2	10-12 pounds (1 pound per month)
3	5-6 pounds (0.5 pound per month)
4+	2-3 pounds (not worth calculating)

This means that it's pointless to gain more than 2 pounds per month. Your body simply won't be able to utilize those extra calories, and they'll get stored as fat.

When it comes to losing weight, there are similar limits you need to be aware of. If you lose weight too fast, you risk burning muscle. And this defeats the entire purpose of losing weight.

You want to burn fat, but maintain muscle mass, because you want to expose the muscle definition that's hiding beneath your top layer of body fat. If you burn fat AND muscle at the same time, you essentially prevent this from happening. Rather than getting shredded and looking more muscular, you end up looking like a smaller version of yourself. Less fat, sure, but also less muscle.

So how fast can you lose weight without risking muscle loss?

There's no magic number here, but from all the studies I've seen, I would say that anything more than 1 pound per week is taking a risk. Plus, in order to lose weight faster than that, you're going to have to practically starve yourself. It's just not worth it.

Alright, that's great and all, but how do I actually figure out how many calories I need to eat in order to accomplish this?

In general, if you're trying to gain weight, multiply your body weight (in pounds) by 18. For example, I weigh 175 pounds, so 175 X 18 = 3150 calories per day. That's roughly how many calories I need to eat in order to gain that sweet spot of 2 pounds per month.

And if you're trying to lose weight, multiply your bodyweight (in pounds) by 12. For example, I weigh 175 pounds, so 175 X 12 = 2100 calories per day. That's roughly how many calories I need to eat in order to lose that sweet spot of 1 pound per week.

In the next chapter, I'll give you a simple calorie counting hack to eat the right amount of calories every day (without going crazy).

Counting Hacks

Have you ever counted calories before?

I did for years. And it drove me crazy.

The funny thing is that I was sort of a "lazy" counter. I didn't weigh out any of my ingredients. I simply eyeballed my foods and made some quick estimates. It probably took me 60 seconds to calculate my calories after each meal.

Most people who count calories do a lot more than this. Most people literally weigh out every single ingredient they eat on a small food scale. But even after years of counting calories "the easy way", I simply can't fathom going to these lengths.

I was already so obsessive and anal about everything I ate as it was. Every day, I would constantly be stressing out about how many more calories I had left to "spend". If I had dinner plans, I would anxiously examine the restaurant's menu earlier in the day, trying to determine how many calories were in each dish I might order. And if it was unclear where we were going to eat, I would be a nervous wreck.

Don't get me wrong, I still think about food a lot

now, but it almost makes me sick to remember how compulsive my thoughts used to be. To be clear, this was around the same time I had the "bigorexia" body image issues I explained back in Part I. As you can see now, I clearly had an eating disorder to go along with it.

The sad thing is that I see a lot of men suffering from the same issues today. Sometimes it's a guy I meet at the gym, explaining his diet and training routine to me in detail. Sometimes it's a YouTube or Instagram star, explaining his regimen to his followers. And it makes me sad. Because I know that thousands of guys are watching these videos and following this advice.

Now, I'm sure that some people can count calories every single day without developing body image issues or eating disorders. But I'm also sure that many of us cannot.

However, as I explained in the previous chapter, you NEED to eat the right amount of calories if you want to make efficient progress. And you need to count your calories if you want to ensure you're actually eating the right amount. It's simply not possible to do so otherwise.

Seems like a lose-lose situation, doesn't it?

Fortunately, there's a solution – an easy "hack" to eat the right amount of calories every single day without getting completely obsessed:

Count your calories for 2 weeks, so that you know roughly how much you should be eating every day, and then stop counting.

This allows you to make sure you're eating roughly the right amount of food to pack on mass (or shred fat) efficiently. And it allows you to do so without having to track your diet every single day for the rest of your life.

But how accurate is this method?

Obviously, it's not as precise as counting your calories every single day. However, even with daily tracking, you're never going to be 100% accurate. There's simply too much room for error, between overestimating food amounts, underestimating food amounts, and forgetting to count specific ingredients.

After counting your calories for two weeks, you will have a good "feel" for how big each of your meals should be. At this point, you can give up the tedious process of counting and just maintain your new portion sizes.

If you've never counted calories before, here's a simple way to get started:

- Download the MyFitnessPal app on your smartphone

- After each meal, enter in each food you ate into the app
- At the end of the day, see how many total calories you ate

When you plug your foods into the app, you're going to need a simple system to estimate your portion sizes. Refer to these guidelines:

- 1 tablespoon is the size of a golf ball (used to estimate foods like peanut butter or olive oil)
- 1 cup is the size of your clenched fist (used to estimate foods like milk or cereal)
- 3 ounces is the size of a bar of soap (used to estimate foods like meat or fish)

In the next chapter, I'll show you a simple hack to track your progress and make sure your diet remains consistent in the long term.

Smoke and Mirrors

Have you ever heard the saying "what doesn't get measured, doesn't get managed"?

It basically means that if you leave things up to chance, they probably won't turn out as planned.

For example, if you don't keep track of your spending, you're more likely to blow your savings. Or if you run a business, and you don't keep track of how many new leads you're getting, you're more likely to end up with a drop in sales.

But this principle can also be applied to your fitness goals...

For example, if you don't count your calories, you're unlikely to eat the correct amount of food. Or if you don't track your weights in the gym, you're unlikely to push yourself to lift more weight and grow stronger.

It also means that you should weigh yourself and take progress photos to measure how effective your diet and workouts have been.

If you don't do these things, and you don't measure your progress, then you're likely to end up looking exactly same, year after year.

As I said, "what doesn't get measured, doesn't get managed."

However, most people get this process completely wrong. Most people end up taking incorrect and inaccurate measurements. And this is arguably worse than not measuring anything at all.

For example, a lot of people weigh themselves every single day. Even worse, they weigh themselves at completely different times of day.

You see, your bodyweight varies based on many different factors. Here are just a few of them:

- Hydration (Did you just drink a full glass of water? Or maybe you haven't drunk in hours?)
- How much food you've eaten
- How many carbs you ate yesterday (This affects your glycogen stores as previously explained)
- How much sodium you consumed yesterday (This also affects your water weight)
- The last time you used the bathroom

If you compare today's morning weight with yesterday's afternoon weight, it's like comparing apples to oranges. It's like determining how much money you have saved up by looking at one receipt, rather than checking your bank account balances. It doesn't make sense.

Instead, you need to control the conditions when you weigh yourself. The best way to do this is to weigh yourself first thing in the morning, after using the bathroom, but before eating or drinking anything.

At this point, you're closest to your "true" weight, because you haven't had time to interfere with anything yet.

Beyond this, you should only weigh yourself once per week. Otherwise, you'll be thrown off by small fluctuations in body weight that don't mean anything. Plus, having to weigh yourself every day is only going to make you more obsessive about your diet. And this can only hurt your confidence and self-esteem.

Okay, but how should I actually use this information?

After you've tracked your bodyweight for one month, you will have 4 separate weekly measurements. This means you will know roughly how much weight you're losing (or gaining) per week.

If this number is higher than 2 pounds per month (if you're gaining weight) or 1 pound per week (if you're losing weight), then you know you need to adjust your calories. Eat a little bit more, or a little bit less, depending on your personal goals.

(Side note: re-read the last chapter if you forget how much weight you should be aiming to lose or gain.)

In addition to weighing yourself, you should also take progress photos.

I recommend taking progress photos because the scale can only tell you so much.

Between fluctuations in water weight, fat loss, and muscle gain, there are a lot of different factors that can affect your body weight. Progress photos, on the other hand, will give you a more accurate picture of your actual progress.

Why not just look in the mirror every day?

Because progress occurs over months and years, not day-to-day. In fact, it's easy to trick yourself into thinking you haven't made any progress when in fact you have. When you see yourself in the mirror every day, it creates an illusion that your body never changes, because of how slowly progress takes place.

For this reason, I advise taking progress photos every 3 months. This is frequent enough to keep you motivated and excited to see how much new progress you've made, but not so frequent that it makes you obsessive about your body.

Take the photos in the mirror, with your shirt off. Take one from the front and one from the side, so you can get a comprehensive look at any changes that have taken place.

To recap this chapter, there are two simple "hacks"

you should use to measure your progress.

- Weigh yourself once per week, first thing in the morning
- Take progress photos every 3 months

Doing these two simple things will allow you to accurately measure your progress, and this will help keep you motivated, focused, and consistent with your diet and your training routine.

The Shortcut to Gains

Is your main goal to build muscle or get lean?

If you're like most guys, then you probably want to do both. You want to get bigger. And you want to get leaner.

Now, as we explored in a previous chapter, you need to gain weight to create an optimal environment for muscle growth. And you need to lose weight to create an optimal environment for fat loss.

In other words, it's not practical to try and do both at the same time. This is why bodybuilders traditionally alternate between "bulking" and "cutting". They gain weight and build muscle for several months in a row. Then they switch gears and lose weight, in order to burn off the extra fat they gained during their "bulking" phase.

Now, this process is proven to work. But here's the thing: it's not ideal for regular dudes.

You see, during a traditional "bulk" it's normal to gain one pound or more per week. But as we explored previously, your body is only naturally capable of building half a pound of muscle per week (at most).

So why do these bodybuilders gain weight so fast?

Simple. Most of them use steroids. And this allows them to pack on muscle faster than is possible without drugs.

In other words, traditional bulking and cutting is useless for regular dudes like you or me. In fact, it's actually counter-productive, because you'll end up putting on a bunch of fat every time you bulk. And this means you'll have to waste months and months burning it back off...

So the real question is: can you "hack" this process and build muscle while also staying lean all year round?

Yes! Luckily there's a better option for guys who want to build muscle and get leaner without drugs.

The first step is to cut down and get lean (before you worry about bulking up and building muscle). Why? Because getting lean naturally boosts testosterone.

Studies show that higher levels of body fat are linked with lower levels of testosterone and decreased insulin sensitivity. They also confirm that it's possible to increase your testosterone (and your insulin sensitivity) simply by lowering your body fat percentage. [13]

This is significant because both of these things play a large role in the muscle building process.

You see, higher levels of testosterone (and increased insulin sensitivity) both lead to higher rates of muscle protein synthesis. And this means that you get to build more muscle.

Let me phrase this in a different way, in case that doesn't make sense: when you get lean, your body becomes more efficient at building muscle. For every pound of body weight you gain, more of it will be muscle and less of it will be fat (versus when you're at a higher body fat percentage).

Plus, testosterone levels also play a large role in your sex drive and your overall energy levels.

And that's not the only reason to get lean first...

We all want to look good naked. And the key to looking good naked is being lean.

Yes, you also want to have some muscle on your frame. But if it's covered by a thick layer of fat, you're still going to look like shit. When you get lean, you essentially remove that layer of fat and expose your muscle definition. Even if you're not quite as big as you want to be, you will still look good.

So by cutting down first, you get the gratification of looking good sooner, rather than delaying that gratification for months and months of bulking up and looking chubby.

Okay cool, but exactly how lean do I need to get?

Good question. There's no perfect answer here, but I believe you should cut down to around 12-15% body fat. This means you should be able to see your six-pack when you flex.

For most guys, this will allow you to optimize your hormone levels and look good naked, without starving yourself or risking developing an eating disorder.

You see, the leaner you get, the more you'll have to restrict your calories in order to keep burning fat and losing weight. And once you approach about 10% body fat, this can become a painful process. In my opinion, there's no reason to subject yourself to that pain unless you're planning to become a fitness model or doing a bodybuilding competition.

...Now, once you're lean, it's time to switch gears and build some muscle!

However, if you don't want to gain fat in the process, you need to be careful here.

As I mentioned above, your body is only naturally capable of synthesizing about half a pound of muscle per week... and that's only if you're brand new to lifting! This means that any weight you gain beyond this point will be strictly fat.

So, given this natural limit, you should aim to gain half a pound per week (or 2 pounds per month) in order to optimize muscle growth. This ensures that your body has the energy it needs to synthesize new muscle tissue. It also ensures that you don't go overboard and gain a bunch of fat.

And, as a natural lifter, this is your best possible option. It allows you to gain size and get bigger while staying lean (and maintaining optimal hormone levels) all year round!

Okay, let's quickly review the best way to build muscle without steroids:

- Start by losing weight and getting lean (12-15% body fat)
- This will increase your testosterone, and you'll look better naked
- Next, start gaining weight (2 pounds per month is optimal)
- This will max out your natural muscle growth limits and minimize fat gain

This simple system will allow you to consistently get bigger and stronger. Plus, it will make sure you stay lean all year round in the process!

However, you also need to make sure that your workout routine is optimized for building muscle. But don't worry, you'll learn everything you need to know about that in Part III.

PART III: Training Hacks

Stop Hopping

I made very little progress during my first few years working out.

The first "program" I tried was P90X. It's one of those home workout series where you follow along with some guys on camera. I think it was like 9 DVDs in total (yes, this was back in the day of DVDs).

I did that program for a month or two in my parents' basement, before moving back to Boston for my next year of school at Boston University.

When I got there, I realized that it didn't make sense to do a "home" workout program. My dorm room was too small. And I lived right next to the school's state-of-the-art fitness center. So I started going to the gym every few days and doing random exercises that I learned from P90X.

...That didn't last long.

Before you know it, I just stopped working out altogether. Sure, I still played pickup basketball a few times per week, but I stopped lifting weights.

Fast forward a year, and I was living in Spain, working an internship at a medium size software company in Madrid. My friend in the cubicle next to me just so happened to be an amateur bodybuilder.

He inspired me to start lifting weights again. I found a simple program on Bodybuilding.com and got to work. Well, I also had to find a gym. Luckily I found one nearby that only cost me 2 euros per visit (3 euros after they realized I was older than 16).

(Side note: this was a rundown "municipal" gym operated by the government. It's by far the worst gym I've ever used for an extended period of time.)

After not seeing any results after a few weeks, I selected a new program. But this program involved doing deadlifts, which I had never done before, and my back was KILLING me after just one workout. So I decided this program wasn't right for me either...

This trend continued for several months. I would pick a new program, find a reason why I didn't like it, and then find something new. I got a little stronger over time but didn't see many results in the mirror.

When I moved back to Boston for the summer, I knew something had to change. So, rather than just haphazardly selecting a new routine, I decided to do some research. Rather than just picking something random from Bodybuilding.com, I decided to browse the Bodybuilding.com community forums and see what programs other guys were having success with.

This led me to choose a simple 3-day per week full body routine. I went to the gym every Monday,

Wednesday, and Friday and did the EXACT same workout. The only difference was that each week I had to do an additional repetition for each exercise.

It seems boring, but after only a couple months I was seeing results. Not only was I consistently getting stronger in all of the exercises, I was also building noticeable muscle mass. For the first time ever, I was able to look in the mirror and see some actual changes.

That's when I learned the most important workout lesson ever:

You have to pick something and stick with it.

You can't keep switching between different programs and different training styles. This will only prevent you from staying consistent and seeing results. This will only serve to confuse you and sabotage your progress.

This is one of the biggest things that separates the super fit from the average, frustrated gym-goer. The 1% of guys who see results are able to choose a program and stick with it. The other 99% are always searching for "the next best thing".

You see, constantly switching up your workouts is a huge distraction. You're constantly worrying that your new workout isn't "working" – and this leads to frustration, confusion, and oftentimes quitting.

Instead, you must find a proven workout routine, trust that it will work, and stop thinking about it. This will allow you to put all your focus towards actually going to the gym and crushing your workouts. And this is ultimately what will allow you to make fast progress.

Think about it like this: if you want to invest money in the stock market, there are a lot of different strategies you can follow. You can play the long game and invest in index funds that simply match the growth of the market as a whole. Or you can do research, pick individual stocks, and try to build your own custom portfolio. Or you can embrace the high risk, high reward strategy of day trading.

All of these strategies can work. But if you start to haphazardly mix them together, without thinking about how each investment affects the next? You're going to end up broke faster than you can say "bacon and eggs".

When it comes to working out, the differences aren't so pronounced, but the same principle holds true. You have to shift your mindset from "I need to find the best routine" to "I need to crush my next workout".

Again, all you need to do is find a simple routine that's proven to work. And then you need to stick with it.

Also, make sure it fits your lifestyle. If you only have 3 days per week to hit the gym, obviously a 5-day per week routine doesn't make any sense. If you hate powerlifting, then a routine that focuses on heavy squats and deadlifts also doesn't make sense.

If you're looking for a simple 3-day per week routine to get started, I have a FREE workout routine that's optimized for building muscle.

Go here to download it now:
http://www.howtobeast.com/get-jacked/

Instant Gains

What if I told you there was a way you could INSTANTLY appear taller, stronger, and more muscular... without lifting a single weight?

It almost sounds too good to be true. But it's not.

It's called posture. Have you heard of it?

Almost everyone I know who goes to the gym wants to look better. And almost all of them have terrible posture.

It's actually funny to me. Some people kill themselves in the gym every single day, for hours and hours, all because they want to look better. Yet they don't take 2 seconds to adjust their posture.

Good posture makes your shoulders look broader, and it also makes you appear taller. In fact, studies confirm that we rate people as significantly more attractive if they simply correct their posture and stand upright. [14]

Not only that, but they've even done studies that investigate how your posture affects your mindset. In one study, people were asked to write down their best or worse qualities. Some participants were asked to do this activity sitting straight up and pushing their chest out (confident posture), while others were asked to slouch forward (doubtful posture).

Afterward, everyone completed self-evaluations. People who did the activity with good posture were far more confident in their answers than the people who did the activity while slouching forward. [15]

In other words, you're a lot more confident and sure of yourself when you stand (or sit) upright with strong posture.

It's pretty clear that everyone should take the time to "hack" their posture… especially if you're going through the hassle of working out and dieting to improve your body.

Honestly, you'd be stupid to ignore this "low hanging fruit".

Okay, so what's the easiest way to "hack" my posture?

Here are 2 simple steps to quickly correct your posture:

#1: Pull back your shoulders

The first step is to straighten your back.

When most people try to do this, they "puff" out their chest. But this is incorrect. Sure, it's better than slouching forward, but this is bad for your back. Plus, it's impossible to hold this position all day long.

(And it looks like you're trying way too hard.)

Instead, you should focus on pulling back your shoulders. Imagine pinching a coin in between your shoulder blades. This will keep your back straight, make your shoulders look broader, and give you some extra height.

#2: Hold your head high

The second step is to straighten your neck.

Most people constantly strain their necks and stick their heads out in front of them. This is bad for your spine, and it makes you look shorter.

Instead, you should focus on holding your head high. Imagine trying to "reach" the crown of your head directly upwards towards the ceiling.

If you do these two things, your posture will be better than 99% of the world's population. You will immediately look – and feel – taller, stronger, and more confident.

Now, obviously, it can be hard to maintain this position all day long. You're naturally going to fall back into your old habits when you're tired or stressed out. The most important thing is to catch yourself whenever you're slouching.

Simply notice that your posture is slacking, then pull your shoulders back and hold your head high. Little-by-little you'll re-program yourself to hold good posture by default.

(Bonus tip: If you're sitting down, whether it's at work or at the movie theater, here's an easy way to maintain good posture without thinking about it: when you first sit down, just place your butt directly against the back of the chair and your upper back in contact with the top of the backrest.)

Posture gains are the easiest gains you'll ever make. Don't neglect them.

Stack It Up

Do you look forward to your workouts?

If you're like most guys, then your answer is probably: "ummmm, sometimes I guess…"

Sometimes you're in the mood to hit the gym. Sometimes you're not. Sometimes you need to blow off some steam. Sometimes you just want to "Netflix and chill".

The single biggest difference between the 1% of people who are able to successfully transform their bodies and the rest of the population, is that they're always looking forward to their next workout.

They've found a way to sincerely LOVE going to the gym. They look forward to it the entire day. This enthusiasm makes them extremely consistent. Not only do they rarely miss a workout, but they also train hard and push themselves to get stronger every time they're there.

…And this adds up BIG TIME.

If you don't look forward to the gym, you're going to make excuses for missing a workout here and there. In the short term, this might just mean that you miss 3 or 4 workouts per month. In a single month, this isn't going to have much impact on your progress...

But over the course of an entire year? This is the difference between seeing visible changes in the mirror, or looking at yourself with frustration and disappointment.

At this point, you're probably thinking: "I'm screwed! I've never liked working out. I'm just not one of those people who gets hard thinking about some dumbbells."

But here's the thing: none of us were born to love working out.

Sure, some of us embrace sports at a younger age. But, even then, there are plenty of great athletes who genuinely HATE working out. They just love to compete in their sport.

The key is to figure out how to "trick" yourself into enjoying your workouts.

Luckily, there's a "hack" for that...

In the world of self-improvement, business, and productivity there's a concept known as "habit stacking". Basically, it means stacking – or combining – several habits together. The purpose of this technique is to make it easier to adopt several new habits at once.

For example, someone who wants to implement the

daily habits of meditating, reading, and taking cold showers might decide to combine all 3 of these habits into a quick morning routine. Now, rather than having to worry about finding time every single day to do each of these habits individually, they only need to set aside 30 minutes every morning.

Another reason "habit stacking" works so well is because you can include a habit that you actually enjoy doing as part of the stack. For example, if you hate taking cold showers and meditating, but you love drinking coffee, then you can use this to your advantage. You can make drinking coffee the third habit in this stack.

This way, you will look forward to meditating and taking a cold shower every morning, because you can't wait to drink your coffee afterward.

Okay, but how do I apply this technique to the gym?

Simple. You have to find a habit you enjoy and "stack" it with going to the gym and working out.

For example, I love taking a pre-workout powder. In case you don't know, pre-workout supplements are basically a combination of caffeine and some other good stuff that give you a "buzz" of energy and focus.

When I drink a pre-workout supplement, I get amped up and excited to hit the gym. When I don't have access to my pre-workout powder, it's always a bit more of a struggle to get my ass to the gym.

Yes, I love working out... but I REALLY love pre-workout powder!

Also, I really enjoy listening to music. But I don't have that many times during the day when I can just sit there and enjoy some good tunes... except when I'm at the gym, of course. For me, sitting at home and preparing a great playlist for my next workout is something else that gets me excited to hit the gym.

Here's another example. I have a good friend who works out consistently, although he definitely doesn't love it as much I do. However, he loves the protein smoothies from the juice bar at his gym. So he "rewards" himself with a chocolate, peanut butter, and banana smoothie after all of his workouts.

For him, this is the habit that he "stacks" with working out in order to get himself excited to hit the gym. It's easier for him to get off his ass and head to the gym knowing that he can drink a delicious smoothie after.

In fact, he recently moved and told me that he's been missing a lot of workouts because his new gym doesn't serve quality smoothies. This just goes to show the power of habit stacking.

Now it's your turn...

If you struggle to stay consistent with your workouts, think of something you can add to your routine to get yourself excited to hit the gym.

If you're having trouble thinking of something, consider these options:

- Drink a coffee or a pre-workout supplement to get amped up before the gym
- Prepare a music playlist for your workout
- Listen to your favorite podcast while you work out
- Reward yourself with a protein smoothie after your workout

The key is to think of something that you really enjoy, and then add it somewhere before, during, or after your workout session.

This simple technique can radically enhance your ability to stay consistent with your workouts over the long term. And this will guarantee that you see better, faster, and longer lasting results.

Bread and Butter

What routine is best for me?

To be completely blunt, the best routine is the one that you actually follow.

As we explored in the first chapter of Part III, it's easy to constantly hop between routines, and trick yourself into thinking that none of them "work".

No routine is going to yield you instant results. But any "good" routine should yield you steady progress over time.

So what makes a routine "good"?

Let's make one thing clear: there's no such thing as the "perfect" routine. But there are 2 main principles that every effective routine has in common.

If you find a routine that contains these 2 things, and you stick with it, then you will see results. I like to call these the "bread and butter" of any good training routine.

#1. Your routine should focus on compound exercises

Every exercise you do in the gym can be separated

into 2 simple categories: isolation movements and compound movements.

Isolation movements are exercises that "isolate" a specific muscle group. For example, curls target your biceps, calf raises target your calves, and lateral shoulder flys target the lateral head of your deltoids (aka the middle of your shoulder).

Compounds movements, on the other hand, are exercises that simultaneously work multiple muscle groups. For example, squats target your quads, hamstrings, and glutes. The bench press targets your chest, shoulders, and triceps. And the pull-ups targets your back and biceps.

Because compound movements involve multiple muscle groups all at once, they allow you to use more weight. For example, you can use a lot more weight for your bench press than you can use for a tricep extension or chest fly.

This produces greater stress in all of the muscles involved and ultimately this leads to faster muscle growth and increased strength development.

Compound exercises also more closely mimic real life movements. For example, squatting will improve your ability to jump or push a heavy object and pull-ups will improve your ability to pull yourself up or pull a heavy object.

If you play sports, getting stronger in compound

movements will improve your performance on the field. And, if you don't, it will still improve your ability to perform strenuous tasks.

For all of these reasons, you want to make sure that your workouts focus on compound movements. Sure, they can also include some isolation movements as well. But you should be starting off all of your workouts with big movements like squats, deadlifts, presses, or rows. The smaller movements like curls and tricep extensions should be saved for the end of the workout when you don't have as much energy left in the tank.

#2: Your routine should utilize "progressive overload"

Before I explain what "progressive overload" means, let's talk about the 2 main ways that your body gets stronger. This will help you understand why this principle is so important.

The first way to build strength is by "getting better" at performing a specific exercise.

Take squats for example. During your first few months of squatting, increases in strength will come primarily from your body "learning" how to squat.

As you perform repetition after repetition, your brain and nervous system become more and more efficient at executing this specific movement. You are able to activate more motor units and recruit more muscle fibers. This allows you to lift progressively heavier weights. [16]

These strength gains are known as "neural adaptations" and they are the first way that you can get stronger.

Now let's talk about the second way: building new muscle mass...

Assuming you learn how to perform an exercise with proper form, your neural adaptations will be close to "maxed out" after a few months of training. In order to continue building strength, your body will begin to synthesize new muscle tissue. [17]

Just like with neural gains, this process will be fast at first (aka "noob gains"), but slow down over time. In order to maximize the amount of muscle you build, you need a properly programmed workout routine...

In other words, you need "progressive overload".

At its core, progressive overload is a very simple concept: just slowly increasing the weights you lift. This will "force" your body to build new muscle in order to keep up with the ever-increasing demands.

But here's the thing: you can't leave this up to chance! Instead, you want a routine that includes clearly defined guidelines telling you exactly WHEN to increase the weights, and by exactly HOW MUCH.

There are many different ways to accomplish this, but here's a simple system that works well:

- Choose a specific number of sets and reps for every exercise you do. For example, 3 sets of 8.
- For each exercise, choose a starting weight that's relatively easy for you. You should be able to do all of your sets and reps with good form.
- Increase the weight by 5 pounds every week. Keep the number of sets and reps constant.
- If you fail to do all of your sets and reps, subtract 10% of the total weight. Next week, use 90% of the weight you failed with and start again from there.

Like I said, there are many different ways to accomplish "progressive overload", but I hope that helps clarify the concept.

Regardless of what routine you choose to follow in the gym, make sure it focuses on compound exercises and includes progressive overload... at least if you want to build muscle and get stronger as fast as possible.

If you're looking for a simple routine to get started, I have a FREE workout routine that includes both of these "bread and butter" principles.

Go here to download it now:
http://www.howtobeast.com/get-jacked/

The Truth about Cardio

Do you actually enjoy doing cardio?

Correct me if I'm wrong here, but I can't think of too many things that are more boring than chugging away on a treadmill for 45 minutes.

Why would you ever do something like that?

If you're like most guys, you're probably thinking, "Because it burns fat, right?"

And it's easy to see why you would think that. That's what just about everybody thinks. Hell, it's even common for cardio machines to tell you that you're in the "fat burning" zone after 15 or 20 minutes of using them.

...But it's all BS: cardio does NOT burn fat.

As we explored in Part II, you burn fat by eating fewer calories and lifting weights. Eating fewer calories gives your body a reason to lose weight, and lifting weights gives your body a reason to maintain your muscle (and therefore burn body fat for energy).

Now, if done right, cardio can help you burn fat. But before I explain that, let's define what cardio means in the first place....

Cardio – or aerobic exercise – is exercise that uses oxygen to break down fats and carbohydrates to provide your body energy. This energy is primarily used to fuel low to moderate intensity exercise that takes place over an extended period of time.

In other words, cardio is any exercise that keeps your heart rate raised for an extended period of time. The reason I want to make that clear is so that you can understand the true benefits of doing cardio.

First, it's good for your heart. By maintaining a raised heart rate for long periods of time, you put some stress on your heart, without pushing it to its limits. This will help decrease your resting heart rate and lower your blood pressure. While neither of the benefits is very "sexy" (i.e. they don't help you ripped) they're both super important for long term health.

Second, it burns calories. If you're trying to get lean, this will help you maintain a caloric deficit, lose weight, and burn fat. It's just important to realize that the cardio is not magically burning fat on its own. It's just helping you burn some extra calories.

So, as you can see, cardio is not completely useless. In fact, given the benefits surrounding heart health, it should be a part of every man's training regimen.

...But only a small part.

You see, studies show that too much cardio can actually cripple your testosterone levels.

One study examined the hormone profiles of a group of men. Before the start of the trial, none of the men were doing cardio. However, over the course of the next six months, the men began to run (working up to about 30 miles per week).

The result? Their testosterone levels "decreased significantly". [18]

Simply by running 30 miles per week, these men experienced a large decreased in testosterone.

And, as we explored in Part II, testosterone levels play a big role in your ability to build muscle (not to mention it also affects your sex drive and your overall energy levels).

This means that you want to limit the amount of cardio you do. If you're trying to bulk up and gain mass, then I recommend just 1 day of cardio per week. Any more than this and it will be harder to maintain a caloric surplus and gain weight.

Now, if you're trying to lose weight and get lean, then I recommend 2 days of cardio per week (in addition to lifting weights, of course). This will help you maintain your caloric deficit, without going overboard and hurting your testosterone levels.

Okay, that makes sense, but what type of cardio is best?

The best type of cardio is cardio that you actually enjoy doing.

There's no need to force yourself to run on the treadmill if you don't enjoy it. Personally, I love playing basketball and training in martial arts, so that's what I use for my cardio.

Maybe you like to go on bike rides through nature. Or maybe you enjoy group exercise classes. Whatever it is that you prefer, that's what you should do.

Otherwise, it's going to be very hard to stay consistent. If you have to "force" yourself to do cardio every week, it won't be long before you give up and quit altogether.

RECAP: Secrets of the Super Fit

...And that wraps it up!

As you can see, most guys fail because they make it very hard for themselves to stay consistent in the long run. They set themselves up for failure before even getting started.

The simple "hacks" I gave you in this book should increase your motivation to hit the gym, optimize your diet without going crazy, and enhance the effectiveness of all your workouts.

Before I go, I want to leave you with a brief recap of everything we covered in this book. Use the following list as a reminder, whenever you find yourself lacking motivation...

Mindset Hacks

- Ask yourself: "Why do I want to improve my body?" Then ask yourself "why" 5 more times. Knowing your deeper motivation will give you a stronger reason to stay consistent.

- Realize that most pro athletes, fitness models, and

superhero actors are on steroids. Expecting to replicate their results overnight will only set yourself up your failure and disappointment.

- Put your money where your mouth is and spend money on your fitness habit. Nice workout clothes and a quality gym membership will increase your commitment and your results.

- Identify all of your physical insecurities and accept them. We all have things that we're embarrassed about. Trying to hide these things will only make you weaker.

- Prioritize getting 8 hours of sleep per night. Losing sleep cripples your testosterone levels and your energy levels. It's going to be very hard to build an amazing body without enough sleep.

Diet Hacks

- Realize that there's no such thing as a one-size-fits-all diet. We all have different goals, preferences, and digestive systems. Avoid foods that make you feel like crap.

- Make sure you're eating the correct amount of overall calories. If you're trying to build mass, aim to gain 2 lb per month. If you're trying to get lean, aim to lose 1 lb per week.

- Download the MyFitnessPal app and count your calories for 2 weeks, then stop. This way you can make sure you're eating the right amount, without developing an eating disorder.

- Track your progress by weighing yourself once per week, first thing in the morning. Also, take progress photos every 3 months so you can actually see your results.

- Before you worry about building muscle, get lean. This optimizes your testosterone levels. Once you can see your six-pack while flexing, switch gears and start gaining weight.

Training Hacks

- Pick a workout routine and stick with it. Rather than worrying about finding the perfect routine (which doesn't exist), focus on crushing your next workout in the gym.

- Make yourself look taller, more muscular, and more confident by fixing your posture. Catch yourself whenever you're slouching, then draw your shoulders back and hold your head high.

- Use "habit stacking" to increase your motivation to hit the gym. Find something you enjoy (like a pre-workout coffee or post-workout smoothie) to get yourself excited to work out.

- Make sure your workout routine is focused on compound exercises. Also, make sure your workout routine uses "progressive overload" and forces you to get stronger.

- Find cardio you enjoy doing (like martial arts, rec sports, or cycling). Also, make sure you don't do too much cardio or it will cripple your testosterone levels (1-2 days per week is sufficient).

Your Next Step

There's no doubt in my mind that you're well on your way to building a ripped body that drops panties and commands respect!

But here's the thing...

The techniques in this book are only effective if you actually do them!

That's why I created a simple step-by-step program to help you get jacked fast... without steroids, good genetics, or wasting sh*tloads of time in the gym.

It's called Beast Mode Bulking, and you get an exclusive discount for being a book reader.

>>> Go HERE to Learn More and Get Beast Mode Bulking Now:

http://www.beastmodebulking.com

Can You Do Me a Favor?

Thanks for checking out my book.

I'm confident you will build a lean, jacked body if you follow what's written inside. But before you go, I have one small favor to ask...

Would you take 60 seconds and write a quick blurb about this book on Amazon?

Reviews are the best way for independent authors (like me) to get noticed, sell more books, and spread my message to as many people as possible. I also read every review and use the feedback to write future revisions – and future books, even.

Just navigate to the book's page on Amazon in order to leave a review.

Thank you – I really appreciate your support.

My Other Books

If you enjoyed this book, you'll definitely want to read my others. Click here to check them out:

http://www.howtobeast.com/my-books

About the Author

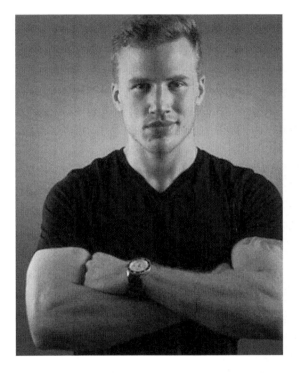

David de las Morenas is a bestselling author, certified strength coach, and the founder of **www.HowToBeast.com** – a popular website for men who want to build confidence, build muscle, and unleash their inner beast!

References

1. Vallerand, Robert J., and Robert Blssonnette. "Intrinsic, extrinsic, and amotivational styles as predictors of behavior: A prospective study." Journal of personality 60.3 (1992): 599-620.

2. Austen, Ian. "Report Describes How Lance Armstrong and His Team Eluded Doping Tests." NYTimes.com. The New York Times Company, 11 Oct. 2012.

3. Gomez, Pedro. "Canseco Says MLB Facing Bigger Issue." ESPN.com. ESPN Internet Ventures, 30 July 2009.

4. Lukac, Michael. "Bulls' Derrick Rose: NBA Has a Steroids Problem." IBTimes.com. IBT Media Inc, 22 May 2011.

5. Green, Will. "Former NFL Running Back Eddie George: Steroids 'very ...'" SI.com. Time Inc, 8 Jan. 2015.

6. McDonald, Lyle. "What's My Genetic Muscular Potential?" BodyRecomposition.com. 19 June 2009.

7. Okada, Erica Mina, and Stephen J. Hoch. "Spending time versus spending money." Journal of consumer research 31.2 (2004): 313-323.

8. Pine, Karen. Mind What You Wear: The Psychology of Fashion. Amazon Digital Services, 2014.

9. Lorenzo, I., et al. "Effect of total sleep deprivation on reaction time and waking EEG activity in man." SLEEP-NEW YORK- 18 (1995): 346-346.

10. Leproult, Rachel, and Eve Van Cauter. "Effect of 1 week of sleep restriction on testosterone levels in young healthy men." Jama 305.21 (2011): 2173-2174.

11. Lane, Amy R., Joseph W. Duke, and Anthony C. Hackney. "Influence of dietary carbohydrate intake on the free testosterone: cortisol ratio responses to short-term intensive exercise training." European journal of applied physiology 108.6 (2010): 1125-1131.

12. Faires VM. Thermodynamics. New York, NY: Macmillan, 1967.

13. Kelly, D. M., and T. H. Jones. "Testosterone and obesity." Obesity Reviews 16.7 (2015): 581-606.

14. Osborn, Don R. "Beauty is as Beauty Does?: Makeup and Posture Effects on Physical Attractiveness Judgments1." Journal of Applied Social Psychology 26.1 (1996): 31-51.

15. Briñol, Pablo, Richard E. Petty, and Benjamin Wagner. "Body posture effects on self-evaluation: A self-validation approach." European Journal of Social

Psychology 39.6 (2009): 1053-1064.

16. Gabriel, David A., Gary Kamen, and Gail Frost. "Neural adaptations to resistive exercise." Sports Medicine 36.2 (2006): 133-149.

17. Moritani, Toshio. "Neural factors versus hypertrophy in the time course of muscle strength gain." American Journal of Physical Medicine & Rehabilitation 58.3 (1979): 115-130.

18. WHEELER, GARRY D., et al. "Endurance Training Decreases Serum Testosterone Levels in Men without Change in Luteinizing Hormone Pulsatile Release*." The Journal of Clinical Endocrinology & Metabolism 72.2 (1991): 422-425.

Made in the USA
Lexington, KY
25 February 2017